I0115359

ISBN 0-9716585-1-X

© 2004 by Mel Angelo Ona,
Published by ONA New Body – New Life, Inc.

All rights reserved.

Printed in the United States of America.

The author, advisor, and publisher shall have neither liability nor
responsibility to any person or entity with respect to any loss or
damage caused or alleged to be caused directly or indirectly by the
nutrition, exercise, and supplementation information contained in
this book.

This book is not intended as a substitute for medical advice.
Always consult a physician before beginning any nutrition,
supplementation, and/or exercise program.

Information contained in this work has been obtained by the author
from sources believed to be reliable and from personal experience.
The author and publisher, for any information contained herein,
assume no liability.

The topics addressed and the ideas expressed in this book are the
subject of debate among nutritional researchers and professionals,
and the author is solely responsible for the contents of this book.

The Food and Drug Administration (FDA) has not evaluated the
statements made about the supplements described throughout this
book. The products described are not intended to diagnose, treat,
cure or prevent any disease.

No portion of this book may be reprinted or reproduced without
written permission from the publisher.

Book cover and logo design: Zoe RajBhandary
(www.creativeinfusion.net)
Back cover photo: Todd Ganci

First Print Edition 2004

1

ACKNOWLEDGEMENTS

Mel O. thanks: God, Mom, Dad, my big bro Eric, my love Jennifer, Dallas & Bailey, Sue Wallace, Khristan Heagle, David and Cindy Schneider, Terry and Judy Strom, Neil Brooks, Nel Stowe, Brad and Marcia Hager, Diane Elliot, Mark and Jeanine McCool, Kyle Brooks, Robert Lorenz, Zoe RajBhandary, Todd Ganci, Pam Brown, Eric Ruth, Matt Thornton (www.straightblastgym.com), Bobby Giordano (www.amacjkd.com), Stephen Whittier (www.nexusma.com), Richard Bustillo (www.imbacademy.com), Fern Reiss, Dan Poynter, Mark Oglia, Sean Hussey, Stephen Rinaldi, Tony Robbins, Will Herman, Steve Downs, Bina, JB, Jay-Bee, Sammy C, Michelle N, Heather M, Cher-bear, Suzanne Chartier, Kevin Collins, Kate Schutt, Tim Ruggles, Dan Robertson, Lisa Amrose, Dave Rash, Randy Doiron, Ramiro Torres, Dave Nadeau, Stephen Shaheen, Tony Wolf and all of my clients who have declared once and for all, *"Hey, I Can See My Abs!"*

TABLE OF CONTENTS

INTRODUCTION

Okay, I'm going to be honest with you about the content and messages in this book. I'm not going to tell you that a "best" or "perfect" diet system exists because in my opinion, there is no such thing as a "perfect" diet.

I'm not even going to argue that "seeing your abs" is the end-all, be-all of every fitness program. I know many folks who are perfectly healthy but who might not have absolutely chiseled abdominal muscles.

And I'm not going to say that my system for attaining visible abs outshines any other system. I believe a system that supports a healthy lifestyle is one that's worth investigating and ultimately applying on a daily basis.

What I WILL say is this.

If you are committed to making positive changes in your health and life, then you must start NOW! KEEP WORKING at achieving your health and fitness goals, and NEVER GIVE UP!

Understand that the guidelines in this book are based on my experiences with

4

helping people improve their health and physiques.

I'm not prescribing a diet/training program per se. Rather, I'm telling you a story of how a person can truly transform without following fad diets or buying silly fitness gadgets.

Also, remember that if you're planning to take supplements of any kind, it's best to stick with companies that encourage scientific investigation and promote science-based strategies for performance enhancement.

Of course, you MUST consult with your physician before starting any nutrition/exercise program.

And no matter what–keep an open mind, maintain a clear vision of what you expect and are convinced that you can achieve, and know that YOU have the power to change your life.

Final note: Write stuff down!

Apply the information you want and discard the things that you don't think are pertinent to your life or situation.

Last thing? ENJOY THE PROCESS!

"Hey, I Can See My Abs!"

This is the very statement that I exclaimed on September 24, 1998 after successfully transforming my physique from fat and flabby to lean and strong in 16 weeks!

I had been overweight (actually obese!) for much of my life and weighed 186 lbs. at my heaviest.

Here I am (on the left) with my dad in 1996:

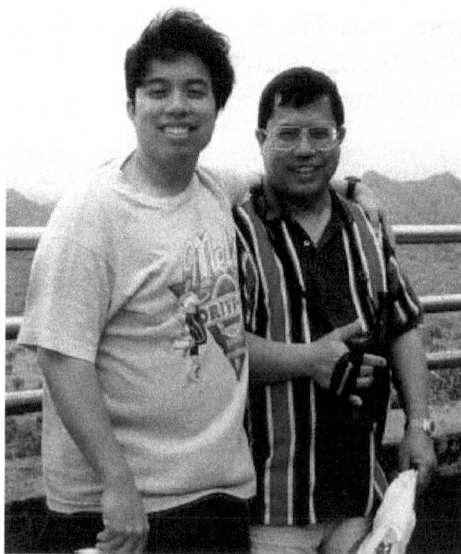

Mel in 1996 (left) with dad (right)

Yes, I was fat.

And of course, I tried every diet out there!

And you know what?

I succeeded in losing weight on every one of those fad diets!

But, the bad news is that I'd always gain the weight right back.

In fact, here's a photo just one year (and oh, about three diets later!) in 1997.

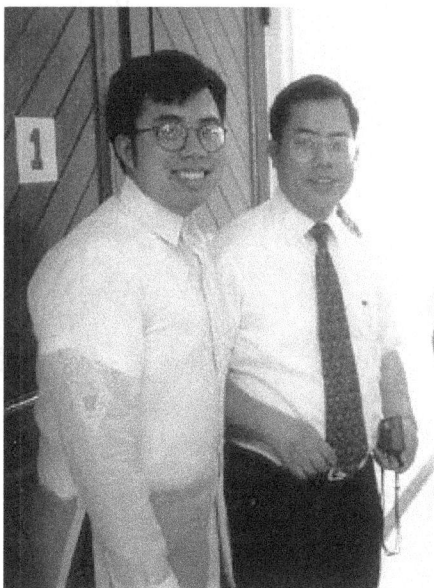

Mel in 1997 (left) with dad (right)

The photo was taken in the Philippines at my dad's inaugural opening of his free medical clinic for the poor.

(By the way, I'm wearing traditional Filipino formal wear, which is a light dress shirt called a "barong.")

I think the see-through material works great in revealing my big belly – wouldn't you agree?!

I weighed approximately 183 lbs. at this time and you can bet that I felt frustrated and utterly convinced that I would never see my abs.

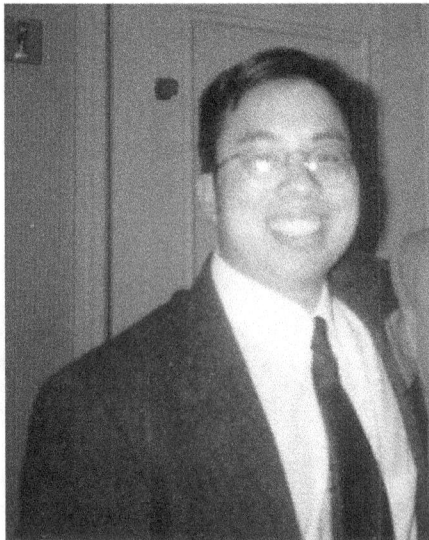

Mel in 1997 @ 183 lbs.

Actually, to give you an idea of what I was doing to "maintain" this unhealthy body weight, here is my typical diet during that time:

Meal One: Nothing! (How many of you skip this very important meal?)

Meal Two: Large chicken parmigian sandwich, 1 slice Sicilian pizza, 1 can of regular soda, 1 dessert item (either a brownie or cookie)

Meal Three: Either a super-huge-portion, fast food cheeseburger and fries or 6 large slices of pizza or a combo at times!

Water intake: minimal (maybe three 8 oz. glasses per day if that!)

Vegetable/Fruit intake: None or maybe some shredded lettuce on my fast-food burger! Oh, and I'd count the fries (potato) as a vegetable too!

I'd continue to "snack" from dinner until bedtime on assorted goodies like chips or leftovers from previous meals.

Here's the nutrition profile of my "Pre-ab" diet:

Total calories: 3,000 calories

Protein: 140 grams
Carbs: 250 grams
Fat: 160 grams

Water: 24 oz. per day (~ three 8 oz. glasses)

Supplements: none

Training/Exercise: none or very sporadic

So what exactly made me change my ways?

Pain!

Pain prompted me to make a life-altering decision to stop eating junk and lying around and start eating nutritiously and exercising consistently. I was hurting my health and I was hurting inside.

I felt more and more disgusted with myself every time I tried a new diet and failed to keep the weight off.

Well, that pain and angst I felt inside also drove me to make a permanent change: a positive change...a change that would absolutely transform me inside and out. A change that has brought this book to you and shares my positive health message today.

This book tells a story. Simply, it's a transformation story. It's about a journey through fat loss and muscle gain.

Don't get me wrong here. I'm not going to say that you've got to "see your abs" to be a success.

Rather, I believe that if you lose excess fat weight and feel great throughout the process, then you ARE a success!

The "seeing my abs" part of the equation is merely a pleasant "bonus" that helps give you a boost of confidence in knowing that you have the ultimate power to change your body and life!

And keep this in mind as you read this book: *If I could change my body and transform my life after countless failed diets – then YOU CAN TOO!*

Mel's "Before" photo in May 1998

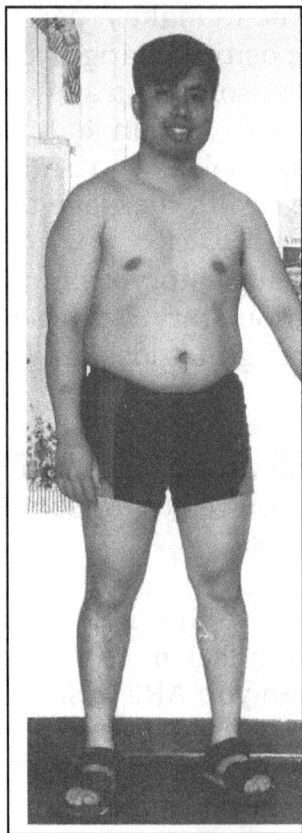

Bodyweight: 176 lbs.
Body Fat Percent: 31%
Abdominal measurement: 40 inches
Body Mass Index (BMI): 30 (Obese category)

By September 1998 (just 16 weeks later) I was flying high! I had developed a new, lean physique and I was feeling on top of the world!

Hey, I could see my abs!

Mel's "After" photo on September 24, 1998

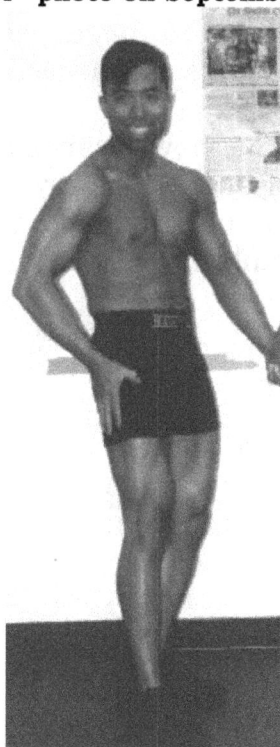

Bodyweight: 145 lbs.
Body Fat Percent: 10%
Abdominal measurement: 30 inches
Body Mass Index (BMI): 25 (Overweight category)

"Hey, What Happened To My Abs?!"

Three months after I achieved the body of my dreams, my girlfriend of over two years dumped me and my healthful habits began to unwind.

I slowly slipped back to my old habits of overeating and this caused me to gain back some of that lost fat weight.

It amazes me how it can take only a fraction of time to destroy something that took a long time and dedicated effort to build.

I suppose that's why "yo-yo" dieting is so common.

Truly, it is absolutely crucial to make a lifestyle change and commit to eating right, exercising consistently, and supplementing smart on a DAILY basis once you transform your physique to healthy and lean.

So, here's my second "before" picture
(January 1, 1999):

DAY ONE

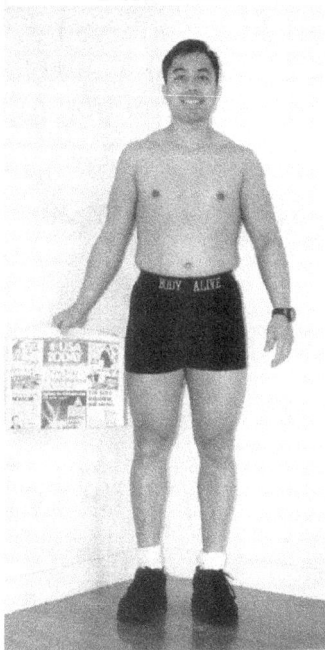

January 1, 1999
158 pounds at 14.5% Body Fat

From the end of September 1998 to the
beginning of 1999, my emotional
weakness and vulnerability simply
distracted me and I failed to follow
through with the actions that had
previously helped me get into the best
shape of my life.

But, you know what?

15

A remarkable thing happened!

Once I got motivated (again!) and plugged in the same healthful habits that I originally adhered to during my 16-week change, I was able to make a startling transformation in merely 28 days!

DAY 28

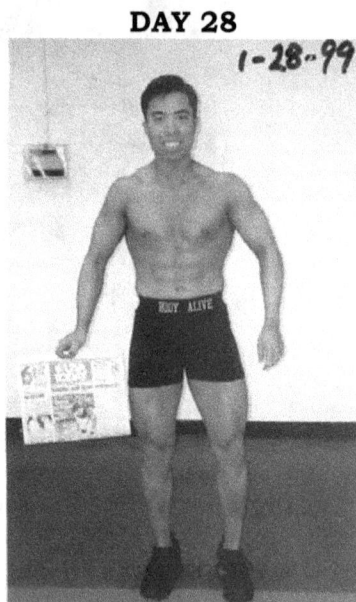

January 28, 1999
151 lbs. at 9.1% Body Fat

That's right, in ONLY FOUR WEEKS; I was able to achieve a leaner and stronger physique than my original transformation, which had taken SIXTEEN WEEKS (i.e. four months)!

Yes, that's right – no hype here!

No picture tricks either, folks!

Completely documented,
unadulterated, absolutely honest truth!

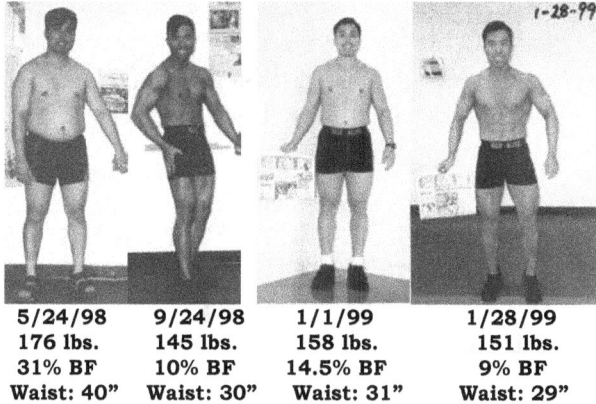

5/24/98	9/24/98	1/1/99	1/28/99
176 lbs.	145 lbs.	158 lbs.	151 lbs.
31% BF	10% BF	14.5% BF	9% BF
Waist: 40"	Waist: 30"	Waist: 31"	Waist: 29"

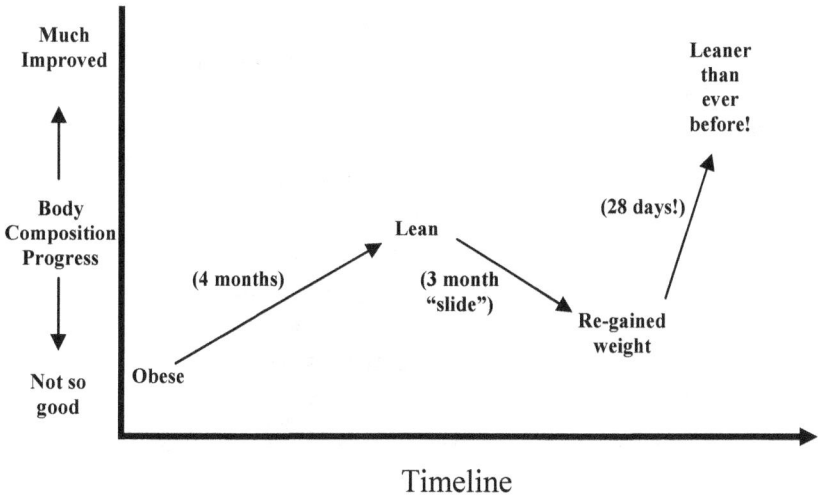

17

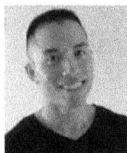

(BODY)BUILDING
FOUNDATIONS

So, my first transformation had laid down the foundation of new muscle mass that allowed me to burn more calories and fat the second time I followed my controlled nutrition and training plan.

The fact is, the more muscle that you have, the more calories you burn. (You'll hear me say this quite a bit...'cause it's absolutely true!)

That's why you've got to train hard to build muscle while losing fat. This is the secret to staying lean for life – even if you happen to "fall off" the wagon once in a while.

Looking back (I keep meticulous journals along the way!) at my program, I realize now that I was probably over-training quite a bit.

I'd do too many exercises, sets (sometimes more than 15 sets per workout!), and reps per muscle group.

Here's a typical BICEPS workout from several years ago:

Standing barbell curl: 3 sets x 8-10 reps
Standing dumbbell curl: 3 sets x 6-8
Seated E-Z bar curl: 3 sets x 8-10
Dumbbell concentration curl: 3 sets x 8-10
Reverse-grip cable curl: 3 sets x 10-12

Total Training Time: ~60 minutes

Now that's EXCESSIVE amount of training for one muscle group!

Now, check out one of my more current BICEPS workout:

Standing barbell curl: 2 sets x 4-6 reps
Standing dumbbell curl: 2 sets x 4-6 reps

Total Training Time: ~20 minutes

Did you notice the training time too? Plus **RESULTS**!

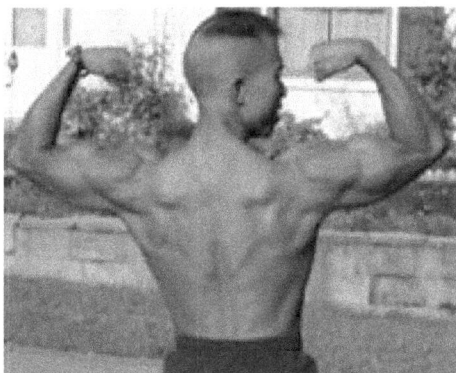

REMEMBER THESE KEY POINTS

Building your best physique does NOT require hours of training in the gym.

Keep your training sessions brief.

Make them intense!

Keep TRACK!

MEL'S SUCCESS COACHES!

I am absolutely convinced that my fitness success is due in part to the guidance and support of some amazing coaches.

All of my coaches have helped me reach the next level of achievement by challenging me to "step-up" and never stop moving towards fulfilling my dreams.

One of my more recent coaches is **Jeff Willet**:

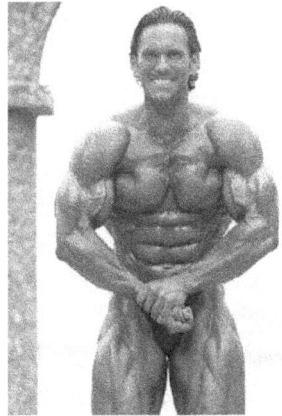

He's an internationally ranked, natural, drug-free bodybuilding champion:

Jeff is an inspirational guy and his own journey is nothing short of awesome!

I've enjoyed working with Jeff because of his ability to instantly spot my weaknesses and change them into opportunities for growth.

Sure, I may already know how to achieve lean elite levels. Of course, I'll continue learning about nutrition, training, supplementation and reviewing the latest scientific research on body composition.

And granted I'll always try to help others achieve their own personal fitness transformations.

BUT, I still find that having a coach is TREMENDOUSLY BENEFICIAL and SYNERGISTIC!

A coach, like Jeff, will help me apply what I know to achieve great things.

Jeff doesn't just "pep" talk me though.

He CHALLENGES me with questions about why I'm doing what I'm doing.

He keeps me accountable and it works wonders for my mental focus and physique progress.

Go find yourself a coach to mentor you!

You'll save effort, time, and a whole lot of pain if your coach practices what he or she preaches.

After all, I think that an outstanding
C.O.A.C.H. –

Commits to your constant progress
and...
Offers outstanding, profound
knowledge and distinctions, which
are immediately...
Applicable and appropriate to you,
and...
Conducts him or herself candidly
and compassionately with...
Highest levels of professionalism,
honesty, and integrity

Jeff is a true leader in the fitness
coaching field and I feel deeply
fortunate to be associated with him, his
vision, and his unrelenting pursuit for
spreading health and fitness excellence
to the masses.

23

NUTRITION NOTES

Okay, now, the point of this book is not to preach at you and tell you what I believe the "perfect" diet is for seeing your abs (i.e. getting lean!).

In fact, there's really no such thing as the "perfect" diet.

The *Law of Individual Differences* means that everyone responds to things in a unique way.

You can give 10 different folks the same diet and training plan and I'll bet that each one gets some variation of results.

One person might lose 5 pounds in one week and another might actually gain weight!

So, with that said, I will simply offer you my tried and true tips for getting me lean (i.e. seeing my abs!) and keeping me healthy.

After all, it should always be about health first.

Looking good but feeling bad is not acceptable!

The goal is to see your abs (lose the fat, build the muscle) but NOT at the expense of health!

Got it?

Good!

Now, here are my tried and true tips for seeing your abs AND staying healthy (by the way, we believe that HEALTH IS FIRST – Consult your doctor before beginning a nutrition/exercise program!):

1. Nutrition is Number One.

Let's face it, you can do thousands of crunches and spend hours at the gym, however, if you fail to manage your nutrition plan on a consistent (DAILY) basis, then you're planning to fail!

You've got to learn how to manage your calories.

Quick review:
Protein has 4 calories per gram
Carbohydrate has 4 calories per gram
Fat has 9 calories per gram

No matter what diet you end up doing, as long as you are burning more calories than you are taking in (i.e. eating food and/or drinking liquid) you will ultimately lose weight.

Losing weight pretty much works by one simple mechanism: **caloric restriction**.

Calories in vs. calories out.

Learn how to manipulate this equation.

Live this equation.

Embed it in your consciousness.

You don't need a Ph.D. to understand that cutting your calories will help you lose weight.

Cutting calories AND increasing your physical activity is the BEST combination for losing weight and keeping it off.

2. Protein is first.

Okay, so you understand that if "calories-in" are less than "calories-out," you'll lose weight.

However, the weight you really want to lose is FAT weight.

NOT muscle weight.

As you probably know, water weight fluctuates quite a bit.

Try this experiment for size – weigh yourself.

Now go drink 64 oz. of fluid and then weigh yourself again without voiding.

You should be 4 pounds heavier because 16 oz. equals one pound!

To ensure that you don't lose muscle weight (or water weight either!), you've got to consume enough protein to build your muscle tissue.

Changing your protein sources from fat-laden to lean will make a world of difference in your quest for ripped abs!

The reason is simple.

By substituting high fat protein sources (like burgers and marbled meats) with lean, low-fat protein sources (like whey protein, chicken and turkey breast, egg whites, and tuna) you immediately cut back on calories from fat.

Here are some typical high-fat protein and some lean protein sources below.

High-fat protein sources:
- Ground meats (beef, pork)
- Fatty cuts of meat (beef, pork, lamb, etc.)
- Chicken with skin
- Bacon
- Sausages
- Cheese (full fat variety)

Lean protein sources:
- Egg whites
- Chicken breast without skin
- Turkey breast without skin
- Beef (eye of round, top sirloin)
- Fish (haddock, tuna)
- Whey protein

Choosing lean protein sources is important from a health standpoint.

Research has shown time and time again that consuming saturated fat (fat that's solid at room temperature – like lard and beef fat!) clogs your arteries and predisposes you to heart disease (our nation's current #1 killer).

Change the quality of your protein sources from high fat to lean and you'll make a significant step toward healthier living.

3. Protein builds muscle.

Period.

If you consume a diet too low in protein, you will NOT give your body enough building materials to develop the "shape" and "tone" you desire.

If you train hard and fail to eat high quality protein in sufficient amounts, you're simply setting yourself up for dieting failure!

That's because you'll likely lose muscle mass or at the very least you'll end up with meager results.

The more muscle that you have, the more calories that you'll burn and the more fat that you'll lose over the long term.

FACT: Protein intake is NECESSARY for maximum muscle gains!

A new study presented at the 2003 ACSM annual scientific conference showed that in trained athletes, consuming high quality (whey) protein contributed to significant muscle gains vs. a lower quality protein!

Even if you're not a seasoned athlete, you can bet that the benefits of building a "toned" physique are absolutely helped along and supported by consuming enough quality protein.

If you consume a diet that's simply *adequate* in protein, you may or may not be able to shape your body accordingly.

However, if you consume a diet comprising HIGH QUALITY protein, this will support your weight resistance training (see tip #5), keep you from losing your muscle when you're losing fat, and keep you healthy too!

Of course you've got to eat other foods too: lots of healthful carbohydrates (and you thought they were bad!), healthful fat (the ones that are liquid at room temperature like olive oil, flax oil and the like), and tons of vegetables!

Now, the amount of protein to consume for maximum muscle is still being investigated. Some scientists from their research suggest that nearly 2 times the Recommended Daily Allowance (current RDA is 0.8 grams of protein per kilogram of body weight per day) of protein may be needed to enhance athletic performance.

Well, my collective experiences and my own professional and personal opinions conclude that at the very least, you REQUIRE MORE PROTEIN than the average person if you're training hard and if you want to build your best physique.

Frequent feedings of lean protein sources will keep you in a state of positive nitrogen balance and this state is ABSOLUTELY NECESSARY for muscle growth to occur.

So consume your high quality, lean protein sources with each of your meals, train hard, rest up, keep track and you'll be seeing your abs develop for sure!

4. Control Carbohydrates – NEVER eliminate! (Why would you ever want to?!)

In my book, *Changing Bodies, Transforming Lives – Your Ultimate Guide to FAD-FREE™ Fat Loss*, I describe my simple system for controlling (starchy, complex-type) carbohydrates.

It's called the "4-C's™" fat loss method.

4-C's™ stands for these concepts:
1. Cut **C**alories and **C**ontrol **C**arbohydrates
2. Control **C**alories by **C**ontrolling food **C**hoices
3. Control **C**arbohydrates through **C**arbohydrate **C**ycling
4. Choose **C**omplex **C**arbohydrate for **C**ycling

CARBS TO CHOOSE:
Low glycemic, high-fiber, unprocessed, unrefined carbs (E.g. Vegetables, fresh fruits, beans, whole-grains)

CARBS TO LIMIT:
High fructose corn syrup, refined, processed, high-glycemic carbs (E.g. Non-diet soft drinks, pastries and snacks, white bread, many fat-free items - check the label...I'll bet ya' these items will be packed with sugar!)

The "cycling" part means that you'll consume fewer carbs on days that you're less active and you'll eat more carbs on training days.

Let's face it folks. Life is a cycle: an ebb and flow of progress, failures, ups, n' downs. So, too, your goals and physique progress will often change or need modification.

If you want to maximize performance and progress, then you must **TAKE CONTROL!**

I have found that the cycling concept helps folks do just that!

I believe that active people should consume MORE carbohydrates because carbohydrates are your main source for energy.

Plus, your brain needs carbs (i.e. glucose, the simplest form of carbohydrate) and your muscles benefit from carbs in the form of glycogen storage.

I believe that you can use carbs as a powerful tool for maximizing your training results. This means consuming enough of the right kinds of carbs (unprocessed, unrefined) to take advantage of human physiology and biochemistry in enhancing fat loss, muscle gain, athletic performance, and overall health.

5. TRAIN WITH INTENSITY!

If you train with weights, you've got to do so with absolute focus, intensity, and overload.

This gives your muscles a "reason" to grow.

Remember that when you're training at the gym, you're breaking yourself down!

You're NOT building muscle – you're STIMULATING your muscle and coaxing it to grow.

It's what you do before and after you train (nutritionally speaking!) that determines how well you shape your body and lose your fat!

Building muscle will ensure that you remain LEAN for life.

Muscle burns calories.

The more muscle you build, the more calories you'll burn, and the more fat you'll lose over time!

Remember, it's about CHANGE!

Positive change!

Permanent change!

It doesn't matter if you're a rank beginner or a seasoned, elite athlete.

Why settle for mediocrity?

Strive for greater results!

Work towards higher standards!

Continually challenge yourself and your body will respond by getting stronger, leaner, and having more energy than ever before!

6. BUILDING MUSCLE *MEANS* "TONING" YOUR PHYSIQUE.

Okay, for all of you who just read the previous tip and are saying to yourself,

"But I just want to be toned and slimmed down. I don't want to get bulky and big"

Well, here's the bottom line.

The ONLY way that you'll get bulky and big is if you fail to lose the excess fat that's covering your "toned" physique.

When you say that you want to be "toned" and "slimmed down" what you're really saying is that you want to see your muscles show.

Tone, by definition, means "partial state of muscular contraction."

When you look at fitness models or people who are in great shape, what do you immediately notice when you imagine yourself looking like them?

You notice – without realizing it perhaps – the **LACK of excess fat** that's covering their arms, hips, abs, butt, and thighs!

You see their muscular lines and rippling stomach muscles. You can't help but admire their functional strength built from proper nutrition, consistent training, and adequate rest.

Now *that's* a toned physique!

Losing enough fat to uncover your muscular shape and reveal that washboard stomach is the main way to getting a "toned" body.

Granted, you might lose a bunch of fat. But if your muscles are not developed, you might not see the shape that you expected.

Thus, you gotta build the muscle! See #5 above (again)!

Working out with resistance (and with intensity) will sculpt that stomach into a work of art!

Remember this fact too: women typically have 10 times LESS testosterone than men, which is why men are more likely to gain more muscle weight than women.

So do your best to BUILD MUSCLE no matter if you're a man or woman!

Muscle burns calories and gives you shape and "tone!"

7. REMEMBER: TRAIN YOUR ABS LIKE ANY OTHER MUSCLE GROUP!

What's the best exercise regimen for developing your abs?

Simple.

The SAME REGIMEN that you use for developing your body.

As you know, I am convinced that progressive resistance training serves as the foundation for shaping and "toning" your body.

Apply resistance training to your abdominal muscles and you'll develop them and the rest of your body into an "eye-catching" phenomenon!

My favorite ab exercises are:
- 3 sets of weighted cable crunches for 10 to 12 reps
- 3 sets of Swiss ball crunches (using my body weight)
- 2 sets of weighted leg lifts

And that's it for the whole week!

Simple, intense, brief – and EFFECTIVE!

8. TAKE PERIODIC PROGRESS PHOTOS.

As you can see from the pictures I took of my abs during the creation of this book, you cannot argue with visual and physical progress. You can never take too many photos!

In addition, you can have a competent trainer use **skin-fold calipers** to measure your skin-fold thickness:

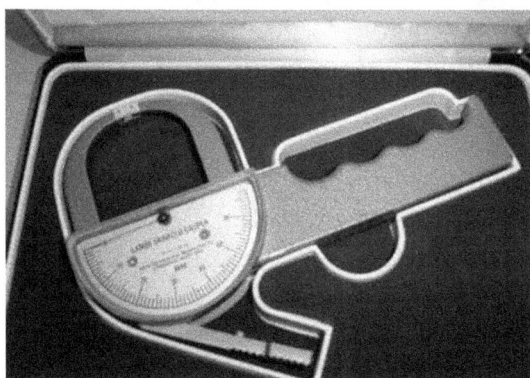

Use a simple **finger "pinch"** (if you don't have calipers)!

Measuring tape:

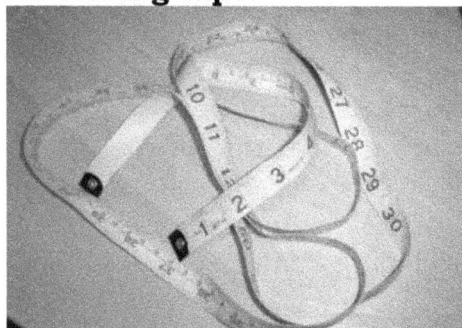

Feeling how your clothes/belts fit and using the mirror to gauge overall progress.

And of course, consulting with your fitness coaches is perhaps the best method for keeping track objectively.

No matter what mode or method you use for measuring your physique, just keep it consistent and notice the trends.

- If you're using calipers or the simple "pinch-test": Are your skinfold sites getting smaller and smaller?

- Are your finger pinches getting smaller and smaller? Compare your "trouble" areas (abs, hips, thighs) with leaner parts of your physique. For example, if you pinch the area on the back of your hand it measures (on average) to approximately 2 to 4 millimeters. How close or how differently do your pinches match up?

- If you're using a tape measure: Are you losing centimeters? Inches?

- If you're using a mirror: Can you see your abs?

- If you're posing for a coach: Can your coach see your abs?

At the back of this book, you'll see progress photos from March 2002 to September 2002.

TOP TRAINING TIPS

1. Building muscle IS "toning" your body...so train to build muscle!
2. Lift progressively heavier weights to build muscle best.
3. Get adequate rest and recovery to help you keep your strength gains from the gym.
4. Warm-up your muscles adequately (but not excessively!) before lifting heavy weights. Again, do NOT fatigue your muscles during your warm-up!
5. Higher intensity cardio burns more calories – so keep trying to improve or outdo some aspect of your cardio training (i.e. more distance traveled in the same amount of time, more calories burned, etc.) at each subsequent session.
6. Keep your lower back ARCHED (never rounded) and flexed tight during your lifts.
7. BREATHE while lifting weights!
8. Spend *less* time in the gym – you can exert more intensity and focus while training that way.
9. Drink copious amounts of water before, during, and after training.
10. RECORD your progress! (After all, how will you know if you're getting closer to your goals?)

My 4-day Training Regimen

Day 1: Chest / Abdominals / Forearms
(Total time of workout: 30 min. plus 5 min. warm-up/acclimation sets)

Chest Exercises	Sets	Reps
Incline Dumbbell Bench Press	3	4 to 6
Incline Barbell Bench Press	2	4 to 6
Hammer Strength Seated Press	2	4 to 6
Abdominal Exercises	**Sets**	**Reps**
Weighted Cable Crunches	2	10 to 12
Swiss Ball Crunch	2	8 to 10
Forearm Exercises	**Sets**	**Reps**
Barbell Wrist Curls	3	4-6

Day 2: Back / Traps / Biceps
(Total workout time: 35 min. plus 5 min. warm-up sets)

Back Exercises	Sets	Reps
Lat Pull-down	3	4 to 6
Seated Row	2	4 to 6
Close-grip V-bar Pull-down	2	4 to 6
Traps Exercise	**Sets**	**Reps**
Barbell Shrug	2	4 to 6
Biceps Exercises	**Sets**	**Reps**
Standing Barbell Curl	2	4 to 6
Standing Alternate Dumbbell Curl	2	4 to 6

Day 3: Shoulders / Triceps

(Total workout time: ~30 min. plus 5 min. warm-up)

Shoulder Exercises	Sets	Reps
Seated Overhead Dumbbell Press	3	4 to 6
Dumbbell Side Lateral Raise	2	6 to 8
Bent Over Lateral Raise	2	4 to 6
Triceps Exercises	Sets	Reps
Lying Triceps Extension	2	4 to 6
Cable Press Downs	2	4 to 6

Day 4: Legs –
Quadriceps / Hamstrings / Calves
(Total workout time: ~40 min. plus 7 min. warm-up sets)

Leg Exercises	Sets	Reps
Leg Press	3	4 to 6
Barbell Squat	2	4 to 6
Stiff Leg Dead Lifts	2	4 to 6
Calf Exercises	**Sets**	**Reps**
Seated Calf Raise	2	4 to 6
Standing Calf Raise	2	4 to 6

REMEMBER: Strength goals (i.e. weights lifted) are matched and/or exceeded each week - MORE strength comes with MORE muscle.

MORE muscle = MORE calories burned = MORE efficient metabolism = MORE fat lost =

LEAN FOR LIFE!

MY SUPPLEMENTATION PROGRAM

Most people know "what" they use for supplements.

They'll pop the latest diet pills, snarf down those candy...er, protein bars, and slug down powders without a care in the world.

However, rarely do they know "why" they are taking them.

Sure, they'll say, "'Cause I'll lose a bunch of fat and look like a fitness model" when pressed for an answer, however, they won't know exactly why this supplement or powder may or may not (usually it's NOT) help them.

So, where do you start?

Several Things to Consider before taking Supplements:

- Ask: WHY before WHAT? In other words, if you do not know the purpose or "why" you're taking supplements then do NOT take them! (My first WHY is always to enhance health and wellness!)

- Determine: WHERE you will be obtaining your supplements from (do you trust the company?) I stick with CyberWize.com (HealthyWize Nutritional Supplements) (www.melona.healthywize.com)

- Plan: HOW will you be taking these to maximize results

- CONSULT your physician first before taking supplements.

- Consistency is KEY!

*Some Recommended Supplements

Supplements from CyberWize.com / HealthyWize Nutritional Supplements www.melona.healthywize.com

*For Losing Fat and Building Strength:
- **Vital Shake** (Blend of whey, soy, caseinate protein; vitamins, minerals, digestive enzymes, and extra fiber too!)
- Fat-burner: **SlenderWize** (Ephedra-free)
- **Vital Stress X**

1. **Why Whey?** Whey protein builds muscle. If you don't eat enough

high quality protein, then you may find achieving your fitness goals an elusive endeavor!

I personally recommend consuming 1 or 2 scoops of **Vital Shake** at least two times per day: especially before and immediately after intense training. You may also have a scoop of protein with your meals to supplement your protein intake. (Vital Shake comes in delicious Chocolate or Vanilla Berry flavors.)

I recommend this supplement for actively training athletes, busy folks, or weekend warriors who might need a quick, low-calorie snack.

2. **SlenderWize** is an ephedra-free, proprietary formula of amino acids, herbs, and specific minerals that promote increased energy, appetite suppression and may help you burn more calories throughout the day. The herbal ingredients are designed to give you an energy boost without the jitters and without dangerous adverse side effects. (Consult your physician before starting a supplementation program.)

3. **Vital Stress X** assists with recuperation and reduction of stress through the reduction of the "stress hormone," cortisol. This incredible supplement contains 'adaptogens,' vitamins, and minerals to counter the effects of daily stress.

*For Energy:
- Fat-burner: **SlenderWize** (Ephedra-free)
- **Vital B12:** Vitamin B-12 is an important participant in energy reactions in the body. Consuming 1-2 Tablespoons of this delicious supplement may give you a healthful energy boost and more stamina during the day.
- **Vital Protein Bars:** These low-sugar protein bars may help give you a late morning snack idea or a late-afternoon boost. For carb-conscious, health-minded folks, no worries – these bars are sugar-free, have no artificial sweeteners and no hydrogenated oils! (Four great flavors to choose from: Brownie; Chocolate Mint; Peanut Butter; and S'mores)

*For General Health:

- **Vital Nutrients:** These multivitamin tablets give you a powerful spectrum of over 125 vitamins, minerals, antioxidants, probiotics, herbs, and concentrated fruits and "greens" for supporting overall health. In my opinion, it's the most comprehensive and impressive supplement nutrient source I've ever seen and taken.
- **Vital Antioxidants:** Fight off those destructive free radicals with an unbeatable combination of 10 antioxidants including vitamin C, vitamin E, alpha lipoic acid, green tea extract, grape seed extract among others.
- **Vital Omega-3** fatty acids (fish oil): Taking 2 to 4 of these capsules each day may have wide ranging benefits in supporting your cardiovascular health, muscular and nervous systems.
- Calcium: **Vital CalMag and Vital Coral Calcium** may help to strengthen your bones.
- General health (joints): **Vital Joints** provides nourishment,

protection, and overall structural stability and health of your joints. It greatly assists with connective tissue recovery from intense training.

For more information regarding the above supplements and nutrients refer to:

CyberWize / HealthyWize:
http://www.melona.healthywize.com

Other Resources:

Dietary Reference Intakes for Vitamin A, Vitamin K, Arsenic, Boron, Chromium, Copper, Iodine, Iron, Manganese, Molybdenum, Nickel, Silicon, Vanadium, and Zinc (2002) Food and Nutrition Board, Institute of Medicine
http://books.nap.edu/books/0309072794/html /index.html

Dietary Reference Intakes for Energy, Carbohydrates, Fiber, Fat, Protein and Amino Acids (Macronutrients) (2002) Food and Nutrition Board, Institute of Medicine
http://www.nap.edu/books/0309085373/html/

These statements have not been evaluated by the Food and Drug Administration. These products are not intended to diagnose, treat, cure, or prevent any disease. Consult your doctor before taking supplements.

(Adapted from Mel's book - *Changing Bodies, Transforming Lives - Your Ultimate Guide To FAD-FREE™ Fat Loss* - **Now** available at www.melona.com and www.amazon.com)

TRAINING DAY FOOD JOURNAL:
(Morning workout - sample format)

Time of Meal	Food & Drink Consumed	
Pre-workout	1-2 scoops protein	
Post-workout	1-2 scoops protein	
30 minutes post-workout	Lean protein source; Carbohydrate Water	Most Important Meals
1-hour later	Lean protein source; carb	
1-hour later	Protein; Carb; Veggie; Water	
10:00 AM	Protein; Carb; Veggie; Fat; Water	
1:00 PM	Protein; Carb; Veggie; Fat; Water	
4:00 PM	Same as above or protein bar snack	
6:30 PM	Protein; Carb; Veggie; Fat; Water	
Pre-sleep	1-2 scoops protein	

TRAINING DAY FOOD JOURNAL:
(Evening workout - sample format)

Time of Meal	Food & Drink Consumed	
7:00 AM	Protein; Carb; Veggie; Fat; Water	
10:00 AM	Same as above or protein bar snack	
12:30 PM	Protein; Carb; Veggie; Fat; Water	
3:00 PM	Protein; Carb; Veggie; Fat; Water	
Pre-workout	1-2 scoops protein	
Post-workout	1-2 scoops protein	
30 minutes post-workout	Lean protein source; Carbohydrate Water	Most Important Meals
1-hour later	Lean protein source; carb	
1-hour later	Protein; Carb; Veggie; Water	
Pre-sleep	1-2 scoops protein	

Some D.I.E.T. Concepts And Notes

D = "Do What Works"

Let's face it folks. Diets do work (short-term). But they also usually fail (long-term).

So what is one to do?

You've got to do what works to support your health and fitness and then be able to live with it permanently!

If you are in great health and you're following a diet that's keeping you healthy, then I'm not one to tell you to "switch to my diet" or "try this one" or "do that one."

Everyone's dietary preferences are endlessly variable and diverse.

You've got cultural considerations, socio-economic determinants, genetic predispositions, environmental aspects...let alone personal motivating factors that drive you to eat a certain way day-in and day-out.

The best advice that I might lend is for you to keep it simple and keep it healthy.

Live **LEAN**: Remember that LEAN protein sources should be your staple as you plan your meals and build your physique.

Go **GREEN:** As in green, leafy vegetables! These are easy to add to your meals and they're chock-full of vitamins, antioxidants, and healthful phytochemicals (beneficial plant compounds). Of course, it's absolutely fine to add colorful veggies as well!

Choose **CLEAN**: As in "clean" carbs – it's a bodybuilder term for limiting consumption of high-glycemic carbohydrates that are highly processed or refined and consuming more low-glycemic, whole-grain, high-fiber, unrefined carbs instead.

And Feast **FREE:** As in eat lots and lots of fruits and vegetables! Why? 'Cause they're healthful and FREE in my book!

Repeat: LEAN, GREEN, CLEAN, and FREE!

(Has a nice ring to it no?)

I = Intelligent Approach

Do your homework.

Keep track.

Make changes when necessary.

Understand that it's a lifelong process.

If you need guidance, here are a few resources that I can offer for support, information, and inspiration:

www.melona.com - A.C.H.I.E.V.E.™ success principles and FAD-FREE™ weight loss
www.melona.com/forum - FAD-FREE™ Fitness Forum
www.cyberwize.com/_templates/healthywize-content/health/index.html - "Health Info" by HealthWize offers comprehensive, science-based health and lifestyle information.

E = Energy Equation

As far as I know, no one has revised the Laws of Thermodynamics!

The first one still applies to the physique transformation process.

To LOSE WEIGHT = You must create a negative energy balance by consuming (food and/or drink) fewer calories than you are expending (burning) through physical activity.

To GAIN WEIGHT = You must create a positive energy balance by consuming MORE calories than you are expending through physical activity. (This one's pretty easy to do for many people, including yours truly!).

You've heard it a zillion times throughout history – and you'll hear it again here...

Eat Less!
Move More!
(And You'll Very Likely Live Longer!)

There's NO substitute for hard work!

No one said it'd be easy.

The ads on TV and marketing ploys that promise weight-loss results with no work involved or by taking some pill or trying some gadget shamelessly violate the rules of fitness success and the immutable Laws of Physics.

Be smart.

Apply the simple energy equation above and you'll begin seeing and feeling changes.

Transform once and for all and you will understand what it means to have mastered this simple equation!

T = Time is NOW...and Take Your Time!

Start taking actions TODAY that will lead you to better health.

Time is precious!

Plan your nutrition to support your energy levels and training gains.

If you're more active, you'll need to consume more carbohydrates for energy.

If you weight train with intensity (and you will!) you'll need to consume more lean protein sources for maximum results.

Don't try and lose too much weight too quickly. You'll be setting yourself up for dieting failure that way! I believe that losing, on average, up to two pounds of fat per week is a prudent, realistic, and great pace for your physique transformation.

Remember, that's "on average" meaning some folks might lose a little more and some might lose a little less fat per week.

Take your time...it's a **LIFESTYLE CHANGE** after all!

If you want to lose fat and "tone" and "shape" your body in the best, FAD-FREE™ way possible, you'll stop making excuses and START TODAY!

Start RIGHT NOW – you will never be the same!

And one day you, too, will be able to declare once and for all...

"Hey, I can SEE my abs!"

MEL'S PHYSIQUE PROGRESS PHOTOS

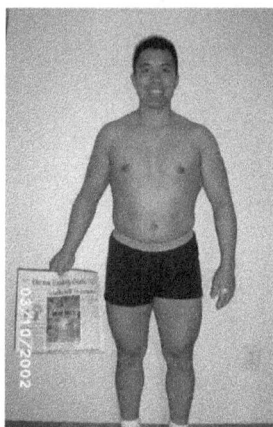

March 2002

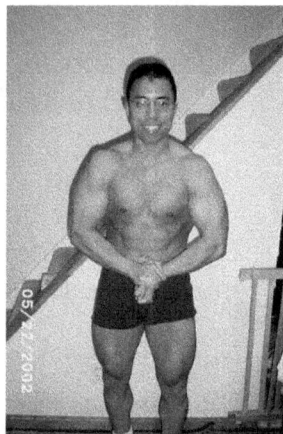

May 2002

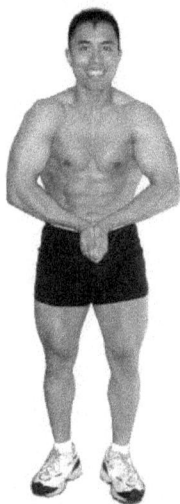

June 2002

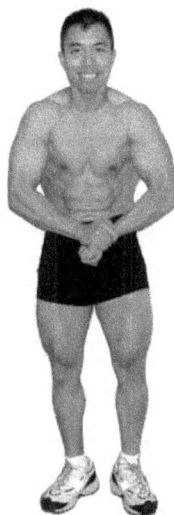

July 2002

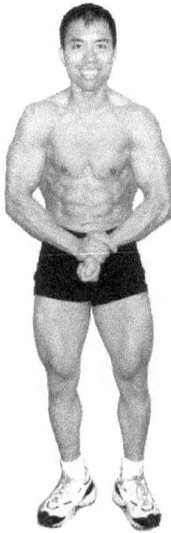

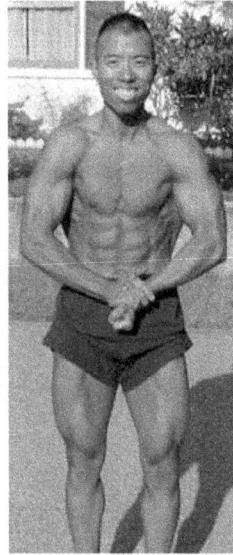

August 2002   **September 2002**

REMINDER:

Don't just settle for "maintaining" – but
rather, keep setting new goals and
continue striving for daily improvement.

Especially if you "slip up" – just re-focus
and re-charge your commitment to
excellence!

YOUR AFTER PHOTO...
...IS ONLY THE
BEGINNING!

CAN YOU SEE THE TREND?

Mel in 1997

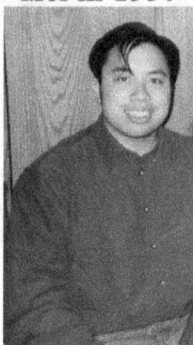

Jan 1997

Mel in 1998

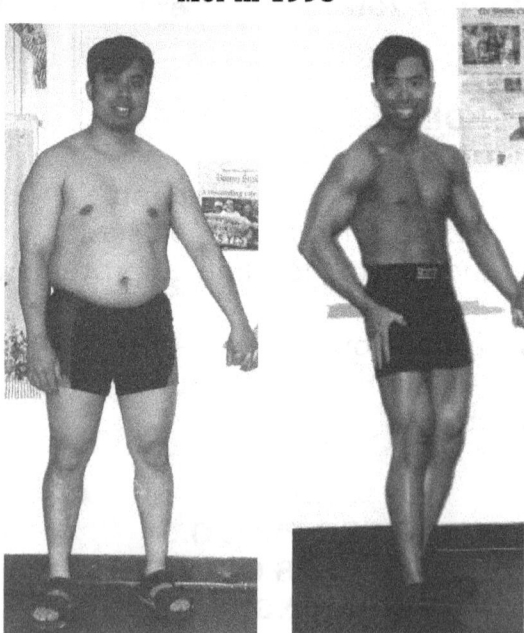

May 24, 1998   **September 24, 1998**

Mel in 1999

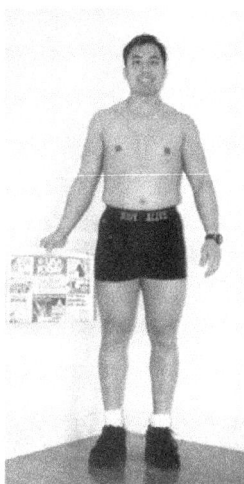

Jan 1, 1999 (Day 1)   Jan 28, 1999 (Day 28)

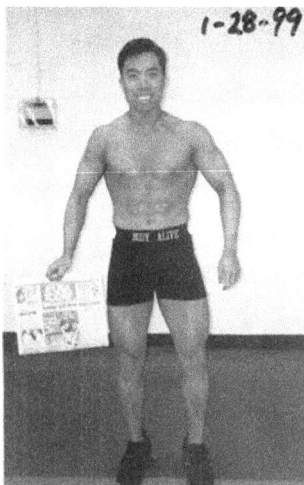

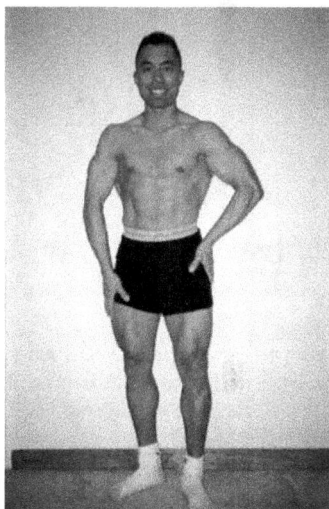

Mel in 2001

Mel in 2002

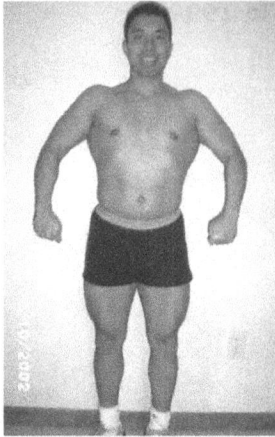

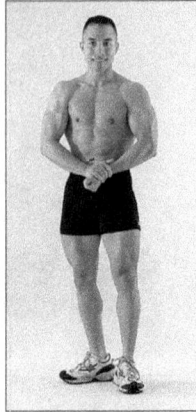

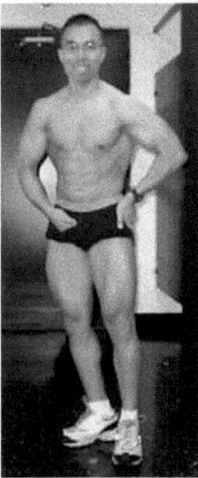

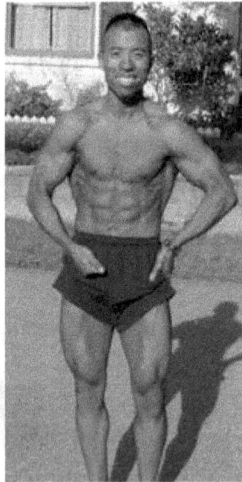

**Lean Elite Shape in August 2002 and September
2002 and still progressing to date!**

If you were to look at my numbers (body
weight especially), you may think that this
trend is the typical "yo-yo" diet syndrome.

My bodyweight "numbers"
1997: 183 lbs.
1998: 176 lbs.; 145 lbs.
1999: 158 lbs.; 151 lbs.
2001: 148 lbs.; 155 lbs.
2002: 160 lbs.; 140 lbs.

Weight loss, weight re-gain, weight loss, weight re-gain.

And you know, it actually is a "yo-yo" type pattern.

HOWEVER, if you look more closely, you'll notice that with each subsequent weight GAIN, I have built MORE lean body mass vs. fat mass.

In other words, over time, I am getting LEANER! Most "yo-yo" dieters get FATTER, lose muscle and become unhealthier over time.

My percentage body fat "numbers"
1997: 33% body fat
1998: 31% body fat; 10% body fat
1999: 14.5% body fat; 9% body fat
2001: 7.5% body fat; 8.5% body fat
2002: 17% body fat; 5.0% body fat

Again, the weight loss is fat and the weight re-gain is mostly lean body mass. Indeed, a picture's worth a 1000 words...or numbers at that!

SAMPLE PROGRAM
NUTRITION / TRAINING / SUPPLEMENTATION

You know, I believe that it's important to "practice what you preach" (and write about!) so I've followed my own FAD-FREE™ Fat Loss Program:

Total Calories: 1,640 calories

Protein: 213 grams
Food protein sources: 105 grams
- 6 oz. chicken breast
- 6 oz. tuna
- 1-cup egg whites

Supplement protein sources: 108 grams
- 2 scoops **Vital Shake** (4-8 daily servings)

Carbohydrates: 152 grams
Fibrous sources: 40 grams
- Broccoli (5 cups daily)
- Romaine lettuce and baby leaf spinach (6 cups)
- Mixed vegetables (4 cups daily)

4-C's™ sources (whole-grain, low-glycemic, high-fiber): 112 grams
- 1-cup cooked oatmeal
- 1 low-carb, high-fiber pita
- 1-cup FiberOne® cereal or similar whole grain source

Fat: 20 grams
- 1 Tbsp olive oil
- 4-6 caps **Vital Omega-3** fish oil supplements from HealthyWize www.melona.healthywize.com

SPECIAL MOTIVATION SECTION

I think that no matter what diet or training plan you're on or planning to try, your level of commitment and motivation may be the difference in whether you stick with the program or fall off of it.

But remember this. Motivation can only get you so far. It pretty much all boils down to whether or not you are willing to take CONSISTENT ACTIONS to get the results you desire.

You can "rah-rah" yourself until you're blue in the face and say, "Yep, I'm motivated!"

But if you don't DO anything towards accomplishing that list of goals you composed, then that list of goals you wrote down is nothing more than a "could have been" wish list.

So, read the next section about my method of motivation.

You'll get motivated for sure - but then GO TAKE ACTION and REAP THOSE REWARDING RESULTS!

Mel Ona's A.C.H.I.E.V.E.™ Principles

Principle 1: A=Assessment, Attitude, Action

Assessment: Success begins with knowing where you are and where you want to be.

You may be making progress but if you have not made an effort to see how you're doing along the way you might be heading in the wrong direction.

Getting your body composition measured is a great way to start your fitness program!

Attitude: My mom always told me "Attitude is more important than facts."

I absolutely agree.

If you have a winner's attitude, then you'll continue to reach for your dreams despite temporary setbacks, losses, or failures.

Maintaining an attitude of gratitude is a surefire way to experience lasting life fulfillment.

Action: If you want to succeed, you've got to take focused, committed ACTION

71

towards your dreams and goals. Your goals are useless without action. Action yields results.

Begin manifesting your destiny...NOW!

Principle 2: C=Commitment Coach, Consistency, Contribution

Commitment Coach: The most successful people in the world attribute much of their success to others who have helped or coached them along the way.

Imagine the best of the best athletes who have coaches inspiring them to dig down deep within and accomplish far more than they ever thought possible.

Seek out coaches who selflessly dedicate their time and resources to bring you to higher levels of success!

If your goal is to get lean, go get a LEAN coach!

Consistency: Making your dreams manifest requires a consistent, focused effort.

Without a constant drive or aspiration to succeed it gets all too easy to settle for mediocrity.

Remain persistent in your pursuit for better health and a better life!

Contribution: You've got to give to live! Give of yourself, your talents, your emotions, and your uniqueness towards the benefit of others.

Be committed to helping others in need. By doing so, your life will positively transform in amazing ways!

Principle 3: H=Higher standards, Healthful Habits, Happily strive

Higher standards: If you want to elevate your life you must raise your standards! If you continue to do what you've always done, you will always have what you've always had.

Reach for a higher goal!

Commit to constant improvement!

There is nothing that stands in your way!

Healthful Habits: Don't diet! Live a lifestyle that supports health, well being, and daily energy.

Forget the fad diets and develop lifelong habits of eating right, training hard, and supplementing smart.

Happily strive: Happiness comes from within you.

Make it a daily part of your life to ask yourself, "What's great about my life? Who loves me? What am I happy about right now? Why am I so special and unique?"

Sometimes being happy simply means being thankful for all the gifts you have and for the opportunity to make real changes in your life.

Principle 4: I=Imagination, Identity, Intensity

Imagination: I encourage you to witness how a young child plays and uses his or her imagination.

There is magic there!

Capture the magic with your own imagination.

Dream big! All things are possible with a dream!

Identity: Remember that what lies behind you and what lies before you are tiny matters compared to what lies WITHIN you.

You are a GIFT of life with unlimited potential!

Share your talents with others. Share your dreams with your loved ones.

Inspire people with your story of transformation!

Intensity: Building momentum towards your destiny and reaping incredible positive health results creates an intense, passionate, and exhilarating experience!

Principle 5: E=Energize, Evaluate Effectiveness

Energize: Learn how to breathe deeply - down in your belly - to experience more energy than ever!

Diaphragmatic breathing cleanses your body, fills you with a sense of calm, and prepares you to deal with daily stresses.

Evaluate Effectiveness: In order to know whether or not you are succeeding, you've got to ask yourself, "Am I where I want to be?" and "What must I do to turn things around?"

Part of creating a successful life requires continual monitoring and evaluation of your results.

Principle 6: V=Values: Vehicles to Vitality

Values: Vehicles to Vitality: If you value health, you'll do what it takes to be healthy.

You'll eat nourishing foods, you'll exercise consistently and intensely, and you'll take supplements that support you.

Keep health and fitness near the top of your list of most important values.

Principle 7: E=Educate, Edify, Evolve

Educate: Knowledge without action is not enough!

Sure, it's important to learn and acquire skills. But make sure to apply what you learn in your life to make tangible and lasting changes.

It's not what you know that makes you grow. It's what you do with what you know and how you do it towards the benefit of others and yourself that counts.

Edify: Build people up. Help those in need. Be part of the team. Conduct your life in a way that mends rather than tears down. You'll grow stronger and gain more courage to face any fear.

Evolve: Everyone has one thing in common.

Time.

You have the power to make something of your life in the time that you have.

Will you achieve great things and live a life that's filled with spectacular health, vitality, and energy or will you just "go with the flow" and hope that there's more out there?

Take charge of your life, demand more from yourself than anyone else could ever expect, and have faith that no matter what, you can never fail as long as you never give up on your dreams!

"Motivation fuels massive action. Massive action feeds momentum. Momentum breeds results. Results are the seeds of Motivation!"
– Mel A. Ona

You can read more about my A.C.H.I.E.V.E.™ Principles in my book, **Changing Bodies, Transforming Lives – Your Ultimate Guide to FAD-FREE™ Fat Loss**

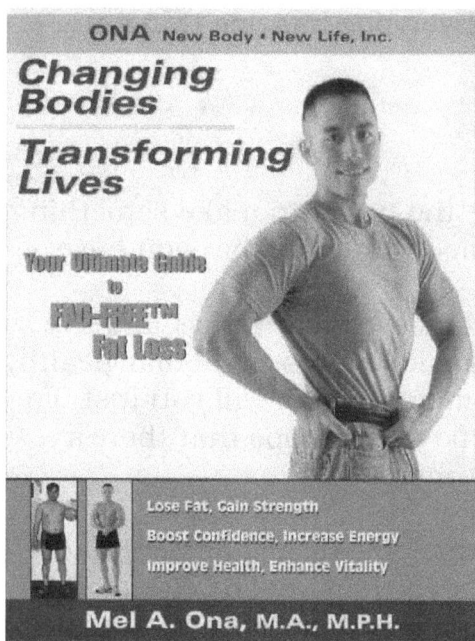

NOW Available at http://www.atlasbooks.com, http://www.amazon.com, and http://www.melona.com.

Your Daily Fitness Journal

(Use these pages to capture your notes, triumphs, moments and memories of your own personal transformation!)

Day:_____   **Date:**_____

Time of Meal   **Food/Drink Consumed**

_____

_____

_____

_____

_____

_____

_____

_____

_____

_____

_____

Notes/Goals/Lessons Learned:

Day:_____   **Date:**_____

Time of Meal   **Food/Drink Consumed**

_____

_____

_____

_____

_____

_____

_____

_____

_____

_____

_____

Notes/Goals/Lessons Learned:

Day:_____ Date:_____

Time of Meal   **Food/Drink Consumed**

_____

_____

_____

_____

_____

_____

_____

_____

_____

_____

_____

Notes/Goals/Lessons Learned:

Day:_____   Date:_____

Time of Meal   **Food/Drink Consumed**

_____

_____

_____

_____

_____

_____

_____

_____

_____

_____

_____

Notes/Goals/Lessons Learned:

Day:_____   Date:_____

Time of Meal   **Food/Drink Consumed**

_____

_____

_____

_____

_____

_____

_____

_____

_____

_____

_____

Notes/Goals/Lessons Learned:

Day:_____   **Date:**_____

Time of Meal   **Food/Drink Consumed**

_____

_____

_____

_____

_____

_____

_____

_____

_____

_____

_____

Notes/Goals/Lessons Learned:

Day:_____   **Date:**_____

Time of Meal   **Food/Drink Consumed**

_____

_____

_____

_____

_____

_____

_____

_____

_____

_____

Notes/Goals/Lessons Learned:

Day:_____   **Date:**_____

Time of Meal   **Food/Drink Consumed**

_____

_____

_____

_____

_____

_____

_____

_____

_____

_____

_____

_____

Notes/Goals/Lessons Learned:

Day:_____   **Date:**_____

Time of Meal   **Food/Drink Consumed**

_____

_____

_____

_____

_____

_____

_____

_____

_____

_____

_____

Notes/Goals/Lessons Learned:

Day:_____   **Date:**_____

Time of Meal   **Food/Drink Consumed**

_____

_____

_____

_____

_____

_____

_____

_____

_____

_____

_____

Notes/Goals/Lessons Learned:

Day:_____   **Date:**_____

Time of Meal   **Food/Drink Consumed**

_____

_____

_____

_____

_____

_____

_____

_____

_____

_____

_____

Notes/Goals/Lessons Learned:

Day:_____   **Date:**_____

Time of Meal   **Food/Drink Consumed**

_____

_____

_____

_____

_____

_____

_____

_____

_____

_____

_____

Notes/Goals/Lessons Learned:

Day:_____   **Date:**_____

Time of Meal   **Food/Drink Consumed**

_____

_____

_____

_____

_____

_____

_____

_____

_____

_____

_____

Notes/Goals/Lessons Learned:

Day:_____   **Date:**_____

Time of Meal   **Food/Drink Consumed**

_____

_____

_____

_____

_____

_____

_____

_____

_____

_____

Notes/Goals/Lessons Learned:

Day:_____   **Date:**_____

Time of Meal   **Food/Drink Consumed**

_____

_____

_____

_____

_____

_____

_____

_____

_____

_____

_____

Notes/Goals/Lessons Learned:

ABOUT THE AUTHOR

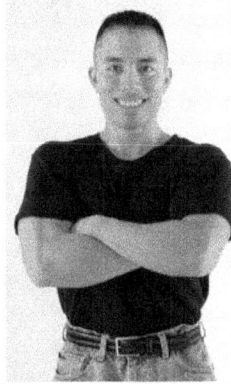

Mel A. Ona, MS, MPH, MA

Mel earned his Master of Science degree in Nutritional Biochemistry and Metabolism with a Specialization in Physiology from the Gerald J. and Dorothy R. Friedman School of Nutrition Science and Policy at Tufts University.

He also has a Master of Arts in Medical Science from Boston University School of Medicine, a Master of Public Health from Boston University School of Public Health, and a Bachelor of Arts degree in music and pre-medical studies from Holy Cross College.

He is the author of *Changing Bodies, Transforming Lives – Your Ultimate Guide to FAD-FREE™ Fat Loss* and President of ONA New Body - New Life, Inc. and www.melona.com.

The topics addressed and the ideas expressed in this book are the subject of debate among nutritional researchers and professionals, and the author is solely responsible for the contents of this book.

BE SURE TO CHECK OUT THESE OUTSTANDING RESOURCES!

www.melona.com
www.melona.healthywize.com

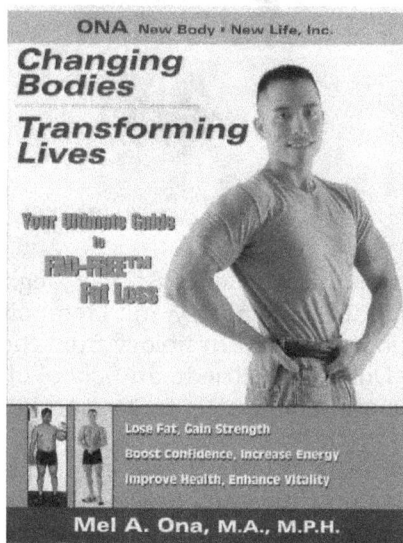

Mel's book is available at www.MelOna.com, www.Amazon.com, and www.Atlasbooks.com

www.ingramcontent.com/pod-product-compliance
Lightning Source LLC
Chambersburg PA
CBHW071339290326
41933CB00040B/1751